How I Manage Diabetes Without Medicine

4 Practical Methods to Manage Diabetes

1. Dietary

2. Physical

3. Mental

4. Spiritual

A Sweet Thank You!

Dear Esteemed Reader,

Thanks a lot for purchasing this book. Your choice of "How I Manage Diabetes Without Medicine" is a powerful declaration of your commitment to a healthier life. I am thrilled to have you on this journey with me.

In a sea of books, your decision sets you on a path to discover the secrets of managing and potentially reversing diabetes naturally. With good eating habits, regular exercise, and the influence of your subconscious mind, you are on the road to transformation.

In a world saturated with diabetes management solutions, you have recognized the power of a holistic approach. Through the pages of this book, you will embark on an incredible journey of metabolic correction, nourishing nutrition, invigorating exercise, and the awe-inspiring potential of your subconscious mind. It is a path to not just manage but possibly reverse diabetes- and you have chosen it.

I express my deepest gratitude for choosing "How I Manage Diabetes Without Medicine" Your journey to better health starts now.

Wishing you vibrant health, boundless joy, and a life free from the constraints of diabetes.

Shamim Ansari
Author, "How I Manage Diabetes Without Medicine"

About This Book

Most welcome to a journey of transformation, empowerment, and discovery. In the pages that follow, you will embark on a life-changing expedition through the world of diabetes management without medication. This is not just a book; it is a testament to the incredible power of the human spirit, and the remarkable potential of self-healing power that lies within each one of us.

My name is Shamim Ansari. I, like many of you, was once faced with the daunting diagnosis of diabetes, a condition that seemed to cast an everlasting shadow over my life. But within that darkness, I found the beacon of hope, the path to wellness, and the means to reclaim my life.

The purpose of this book is simple but profound – to share with you the strategies, knowledge, and experiences that led me to victory over diabetes. The secret to success is to improve the metabolic disorder through dietary changes; As a result, not only diabetes but also other life-threatening diseases can be reversed automatically. In the upcoming chapters, we'll dive into the importance of a balanced diet, the joys of physical activity, the strength of a positive mindset, and the solace of spiritual connection.

I want to be clear – this book doesn't promise miracles. Instead, it's a testament to what you can achieve with knowledge, persistence, and dedication. Your food may become medicine if it is taken in the right way.

Even if you are not a diabetic, this book can be a true guide to keep you free from diabetes. By adopting the lifestyle mentioned in this book, not only diabetes but also other serious diseases can be avoided and life can be enjoyed to the fullest.

Therefore, this book is worth having in every home so that diabetic people can get their diabetes reversed and other non-diabetic people can remain non-diabetic forever.

But before we dive in, here's a quick **disclaimer**: I'm not a medical professional. The ideas and strategies I share in this book are based on my own experiences. What worked for me might not work for everyone, and that's okay. Hence, don't stop your medication. You must consult with your healthcare provider before making any significant changes to your health regimen. The author or publisher will not be responsible in any way.

So, dear reader, turn the page, take that first step with me, and let us embark on a life-altering voyage toward managing diabetes without medicine. Let's begin this journey together.

With hope and determination,

Shamim Ansari

TABLE OF CONTENTS

1. A Million Dollars Secret

It is a universally accepted truth that diabetes is generally a metabolic disorder and is caused by a wrong lifestyle. A wrong lifestyle includes wrong eating habits and wrong living habits as well.

Therefore, if the lifestyle is corrected, the metabolic disorder can gradually be brought back into order. And if the metabolism becomes correct then diabetes will be automatically reversed. There should be no dissent against this inherent truth.

I implemented this natural truth in my life and gradually I got my metabolic disorder corrected. You can do this too.

> *"Take care of your body. It's the only place you have to live."*
> — *Jim Rohn*

2. Why You Fell Ill

Human life is so beautiful. The Almighty gave us an amazing body system with a wonderful mind within. Everybody wants to live a healthy and happy life. Nobody wants to be sick and sad. However, everyone faces health issues and takes medicine. Moreover, some people take medicine as regularly as food.

Do you know why people fall ill? If your answer is no, let me explain the reason with the help of an example. As you know, a car manufacturer knows well which fuel is needed for the car built by him. Some cars run on petrol, some on diesel, some on CNG, and some on electric. What will happen if you fill diesel in a car that runs on petrol, or vice versa? What will happen if diesel, petrol, and CNG are mixed in a car to run it? The answer to both questions is that the inner system of the car will be spoiled and it will not run.

The same is the case with the human body. God created so many creatures on this lovely planet. He decided the food for every creature. What will happen if these creatures interchange their foods? Their body will not digest properly the food of other creatures and they will fall ill.

This means that you fall ill because of eating food that is not suitable for your body. It means you should not eat unsuitable or unhealthy foods. You should keep in mind that your stomach is not a garbage container. Your body is like a holy house. It is a sin to put anything in the stomach. So, intake only pure, fresh, natural, and suitable foods.

The second main reason for falling ill is not doing enough physical exertion. In the absence of physical exertion, the food eaten is not digested properly and calories are also not burnt. Thus, it is clear that if you eat unsuitable food, you will fall ill. To stay healthy and happy, you should consume only those foods that are naturally suitable for your body. Otherwise, you will be surrounded by many diseases and diabetes is also one of them.

The third main reason for falling ill is mental stress. Suppose you take a good diet and also do physical labor, but if you remain under mental stress then it is sure that you will fall ill. Techniques to avoid mental stress are explained further.

> *"Those who think they have no time for healthy eating will sooner or later have to find time for illness."*
>
> *- Edward Stanley*

3. What Is Diabetes?

Its full name is <u>Diabetes Mellitus</u>. It is a metabolic disease that causes high blood sugar in the bloodstream. It happens if the pancreas does not secrete adequate insulin required for the body or insulin is not utilized by the body effectively.

The sugar in the blood is known as glucose. The carbohydrates that we take in our food are converted into glucose. The pancreas secretes insulin. It is a hormone. It controls the level of glucose in the blood. Insulin is essential for the body. It carries glucose to the body's cells where energy is generated with the help of glucose.

The function of insulin can be understood with this example. Imagine that your body cells are like flats in a society and the main door of each flat is closed. Insulin is a vehicle that has a key to the flats. The vehicle (Insulin) carries glucose to every cell. It opens the locked door of the flat to let glucose in.

Thus, glucose is sent to every cell through the insulin (vehicle/key). These doors are known as insulin receptors in cells. Insulin receptors are areas on the outer membrane of cells that allow them to join with insulin available in the blood. The cell takes glucose in when the cell and insulin join together. Glucose is converted into energy inside the cells.

In the body of a diabetic person, glucose does not reach the cells due to a lack of insulin or insulin resistance. Energy cannot be generated in cells without glucose. This is the reason diabetic patients are usually weak, and not energetic. As a result, every cell, every tissue, every organ, and the entire body become weak.

India has the second-largest number of diabetic patients in the world. As per an estimate, about 74 million Indians were diagnosed as diabetic in the year 2021.

As per a report by the CDC- 37.3 million people have diabetes (11.3% of the US population)

"The doctor of the future will no longer treat the human frame with drugs but rather will cure and prevent disease with nutrition."

- Thomas Edison

4. Symptoms of Diabetes

1. Frequent urination

2. Excess thirst

3. Weakness, fatigue

4. Excessive hunger

5. Weight loss without trying

6. Blurry vision

7. Itchy skin

8. Slow-healing wounds/cuts

9. Numb feet/hands

10. Feeling irritation

"The greatest wealth is health."   *- Virgil*

5. Types of Diabetes

Diabetes is primarily of two types-

1. Type 1 Diabetes

If the pancreas stops producing insulin at all, the condition is called type 1 diabetes. The only treatment for type 1 diabetes is providing insulin from outside. The patients inject insulin into the body before taking regular meals. Otherwise, death is very likely. This is the worst stage of diabetes and is generally not treatable with medicines.

2. Type 2 Diabetes

In the case of type 2 diabetes, either the pancreas produces inadequate insulin or it is not utilized effectively by the body. In other words, due to a lack of insulin glucose does not reach inside the cell. This condition results in a lack of energy for the functioning of cells, tissues, or organs. This is why diabetic persons are not energetic. They feel fatigued.

This type of diabetes may be managed by proper diet plan, exercise, and change in lifestyle as well. This is the most common type of diabetes. 90-95% of people suffering from diabetes have this type.

Type 2 diabetes may not be noticed for several years. However, it keeps on damaging internal organs gradually such as the eyes, kidneys, heart, veins, nerves, and liver. That is why diabetes is called a silent killer.

By now you must have understood which type of diabetes you have. I have type 2 diabetes.

3. Gestational Diabetes

This is also a type of diabetes. It occurs due to insulin-blocking hormones produced by the body during pregnancy. It is curable with proper medication.

> *"The food you eat can be either the safest and most powerful form of medicine or the slowest form of poison."*
>
> *- Ann Wigmore*

6. Reasons Behind Diabetes

There are various reasons for each type of diabetes and the same are explained below-

Causes of type 1 diabetes

1. The exact cause of type 1 diabetes is still not known. The body's immune system is supposed to be the prime reason. The immune system fights harmful bacteria and viruses and in this process, it destroys the insulin-producing beta cells of the pancreas.
2. Another cause is genetics.
3. Scientists are of the opinion that Type 1 diabetes occurs due to genes or environmental factors such as viruses etc.
4. If ketone is present in urine, it indicates type 1 diabetes

Causes of type 2 diabetes

Type 2 diabetes is mainly due to the wrong lifestyle and genes. The main causes are enlisted as under -

1. Too much eating at a time
2. Frequent eating
3. Less activity
4. Weak metabolism
5. Mental stress
6. Obesity- it causes insulin resistance. Due to this, resistance cells do not allow glucose to enter into it.

7. Who is at risk?

- People who are overweight
- People living with less activity
- People whose parent, brother, and sister are diabetic
- People being in depression for a long time
- People having metabolic disorders for long
- People having ketone in urine
- People having less sleep

> *"It is health that is the real wealth, and not pieces of gold and silver."*
>
> *- Mahatma Gandhi*

8. Harmful Effects of Diabetes

If the blood sugar level is not controlled and the same is not kept under normal range, it can harm the body in the long run. The below-mentioned complications may occur-

1. Diabetic Retinopathy- High glucose may damage the blood vessels of the eyes. It may cause blindness as well. The problem of cataracts is very common in diabetic patients.
2. Diabetes increases the risk of heart problems. In the long, it can damage the heart and blood vessels. A diabetic person is likely to have heart disease or heart stroke.
3. The kidney may be damaged.
4. Nerves may be damaged resulting in numbness, especially in the legs.
5. It may damage the reproductive system of the body.
6. Feet may be damaged.
7. Can create sexual problems in men and women.

Thus, we see, that a diabetic patient may have to face eye problems, high blood pressure, Kidney problems, high Cholesterol, Erectile problems, heart disease, liver problems, extreme weakness, and low memory.

9. Top Tests for Diabetes

1. <u>A1C Test-</u> It is also known as Haemoglobin A1C or HbA1C. It is a simple blood test that measures average blood sugar levels over the past three months.

2. <u>Fasting Blood Sugar Test-</u> This is the best test to know the blood sugar level of a patient. It is done in the morning after a long gap of 10-12 hours from the last dinner. It is measured in -milligrams per decilitre mg/dl. The normal range is approx. 72 to 107 mg/dl.

3. <u>Post Prandial Blood Sugar Test(PPBS)-</u> This is also a blood test. It is done after 2 hours of having a meal.

4. <u>C-Peptide test-</u> This test is the best way to know how much insulin is being produced by the pancreas. C-Peptide test is usually done with blood samples, but it can also be done with urine collected as per instruction of the doctor. The normal range of C-peptide fasting may be 0.48 - 5.05

> *"Our food should be our medicine, and our medicine should be our food. "*
>
> *— Hippocrates.*

10. What Happens with Patients Who Take Medicines Regularly

Q- Did you ever see a patient who is cured with medicines?

A- The answer is No.

Q- What happens if a diabetic person takes medicines?

A- After taking medicine, the glucose level in the blood reduces and the patient finds his sugar level normal. He becomes happy and starts taking medicines regularly.

Q-Where does the rest glucose go after taking medicines?

A- Medicine reduces glucose levels in the bloodstream. The remaining glucose keeps accumulating in other parts of the body such as in the eyes, kidneys, joints, heart, etc. That is why the eyesight of a diabetic patient keeps deteriorating, the kidney starts failing, a heart attack occurs, pain in joints starts, etc.

Q- How does medicine work?

A- The medicine stimulates the beta cells of the pancreas to produce more and more insulin.

Q- Why is insulin given to the patient?

A- Insulin is given to the patient if the pancreas is not producing insulin. After taking medicines for years, the pancreas stops producing insulin gradually. Medicine becomes ineffective. So, insulin is directly injected into the body of the patient just before taking meals.

Q- After taking medicine for a long time, what complications occur in diabetic patients?

A- Glucose accumulates in many parts of the body. Cataracts are developed in the eyes. That's why every diabetic patient has to go for an eye operation. The problem of high blood pressure develops and heart attacks occur. Kidney failure is also common in diabetic patients. Due to joint pain, the patient faces problems in walking.

Q- So what was the result of taking diabetes medicines throughout life? Was the disease cured?

A- The patient had been taking medicine since the beginning, but his diabetes was not cured till the end. One day he dies due to this disease and its complications.

Q- What should the patient have done if he did not take the medicine?

A- The cause of diabetes should have been removed with the help of lifestyle changes. Metabolic disorders should have been brought into proper order.

11. How to Manage Diabetes

A permanent cure for diabetes is not available at present. However, type 2 diabetes is manageable. Metformin is widely prescribed for diabetic patients. It lowers the level of glucose produced in the body. After some years, the dose of metformin is increased and thereafter, for some more years, patients are advised to take insulin. The dose of insulin also increases after some time.

This is a lifelong disease. Once diabetic, it remains diabetic till death. However, this myth has been proven wrong by several naturopaths. Dr. Biswaroop Roy is also one of them. He claims to reverse both types of diabetes with the help of the DIP diet and lifestyle changes. If food is taken in a natural way, it can become a medicine in itself.

The great nutritional research results shown in "The China Study" by Colin Campbell and Thomas M. Campbell also support the view that if humans keep their eating habits and lifestyle correct, they will never get sick. This book was published in the USA in January 2005. The authors detailed the ground-breaking research results announcing that a Whole-Food, Plant-Based Diet has the potential to prevent and reverse several chronic diseases.

As mentioned above, <u>Diabetes is a disease of metabolic disorder.</u> This fact is accepted in all therapies. It is also true that a disordered metabolism can be brought into order through a change in lifestyle.

<u>The Main reasons behind a metabolic disorder are-</u>

1. Eating too much
2. Eating many types of food at a time
3. Eating frequently
4. Eating unhealthy foods
5. Eating outside foods
6. Eating highly spicy foods
7. Eating oily foods
8. Eating deep-fried foods
9. Eating stale foods
10. Eating packaged foods
11. Eating dairy products
12. Eating many non-vegetarian foods
13. Drinking chilled water/drinks
14. Drinking water just after or with foods
15. Eating fruits/vegetables/grain grown with Pesticides/Fertilizers
16. Doing no physical activity or very little activity
17. Thinking negatively
18. Fear/ stress/tension

> *"Our body is the only one we've been given, so we need to maintain it; we need to give it the best nutrition."*
>
> *- Trudie Styler*

12. How I Manage Diabetes Without Medicine

To eliminate any problem from its roots, there is a need to eliminate its cause. Similarly, if we want to get rid of diabetes forever, then its root causes should be eliminated.

There are many causes behind having diabetes. These can be divided into 4 parts. <u>I did these 4 types of reforms to manage diabetes</u>

1. Dietary

2. Physical

3. Mental

4. Spiritual

All of these four things in your body are dependent on each other. Change in one affects others also. If you think that health depends only on diet and physical activity, then you are wrong.

For example, if you are stressed for any reason, your digestion will go haywire. Due to stress, negative chemicals are produced in the body which spoil the metabolism. Thus, your thoughts are also directly responsible for your health.

Similarly, spirituality also has positive effects on mental and physical health. That is why these four need to be in harmony for your overall health.

13. Dietary Reforms

It is well known that diabetes is a result of metabolic disorders. So, if metabolism could be brought to proper order diabetes may be reversed.

To reform my metabolic disorder, I changed my eating habits. Please have a look at my diet plan mentioned below-

What I eat

- After waking up in the morning, I drink two glasses of plain water or warm water (in winter). I take 2 cloves of raw garlic too.
- I take lemon mixed in lukewarm water twice a week (Sat and Sun) except during the winter season.

(After Exercise and Yoga)

- 1 tablespoon chia seeds soaked in a glass of water overnight.

(Method- Soak 1 teaspoon chia seeds in a glass of water overnight. Mix it well with a spoon and drink it in the morning. There are many benefits of consuming chia seeds. It helps in managing sugar and blood pressure levels.

- I eat 5 peeled almonds daily, soaked in water overnight.

14. My Breakfast

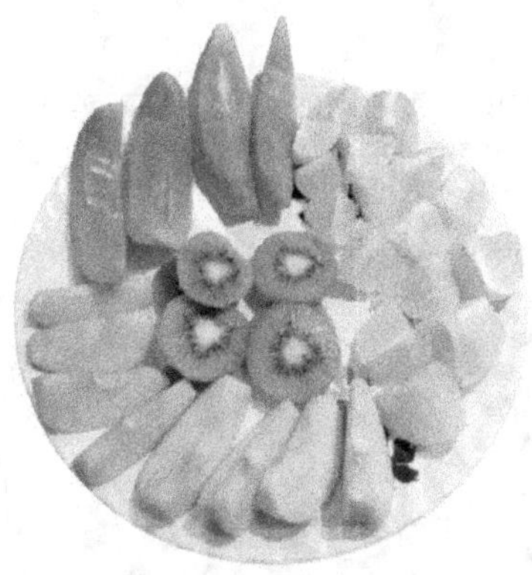

Fruits for My Breakfast

(Apple, Papaya, Sweet Lime, Kiwi)

I eat 650 grams of 3-4 types of fruits like apple, pear, pomegranate, banana, papaya, pineapple, kiwi, guava, etc., whatever is available according to the season. I eat fruits before leaving for my office.

Those who cannot eat all these fruits in one go should eat them in more than one go. Eat only fruits till noon.

15. My Lunch

I usually have my lunch at 2 p.m. My lunch consists of two plates. The first plate contains salad and the second plate contains the regular food of my choice for the day.

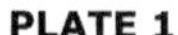

PLATE 1

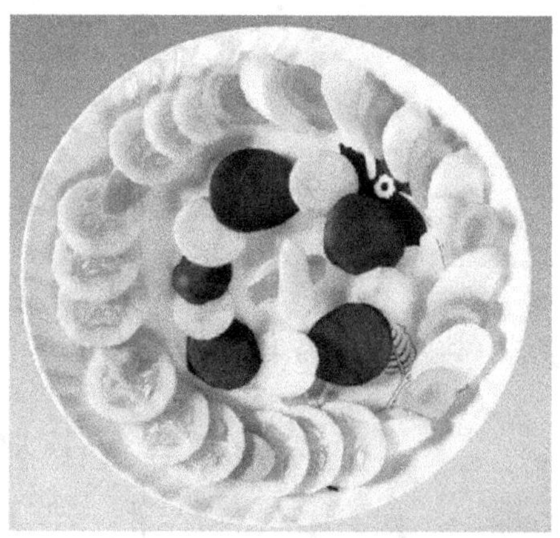

I eat 325 grams of salad - Cucumber, Carrot, Reddish, Beetroot, Cabbage, etc. just before eating Plate 2. You can take items as per your choice or availability.

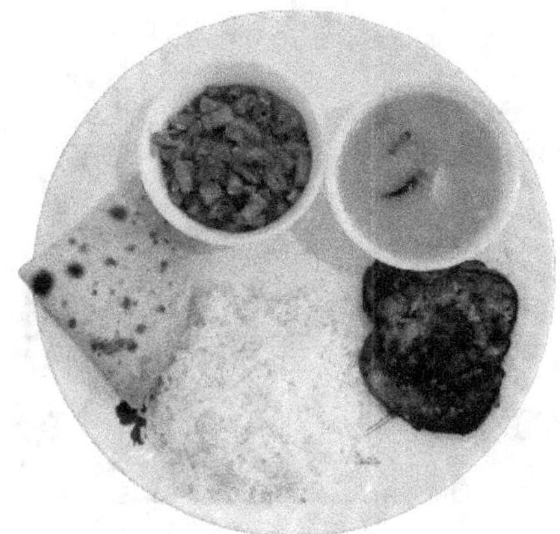

My Lunch- Bread, Brown Rice, Pulse, Vegetable

- One bread/ Chapati made of wheat
- One small bowl of *Brown Rice* (approx. 50 grams)
- One small bowl of pulse
- One small bowl of vegetables, etc

16. My Evening Snacks

My evening tea time is 6.30 - 7.00 pm

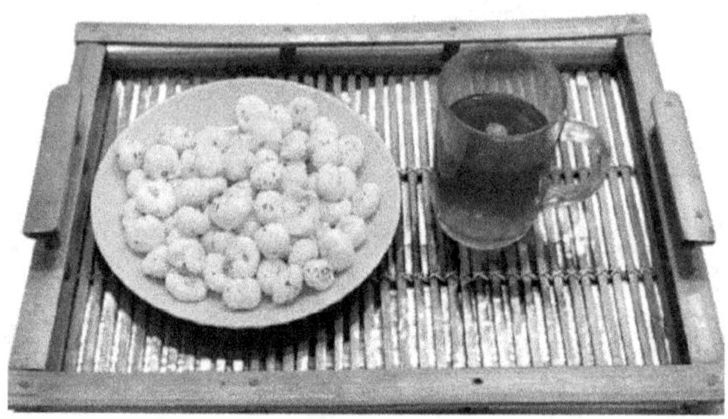

<u>Green Tea</u> –

- It helps manage blood sugar levels, fat burning, liver disorders, weight loss, inflammation, etc.
- It reduces risks of heart attack, and cancer

<u>Baked Fox Nut</u> –

- It is rich in nutrients.
- It is a high antioxidant and anti-aging.
- It may help in controlling type-2 Diabetes, heart diseases, cancers, weight loss, etc.

17. My Dinner

My dinner time is 8.30-9.00 pm. My dinner also consists of two plates. The first plate contains salad and the second plate contains one bowl of cooked Oats or Daliya (crushed wheat).

Plate-1

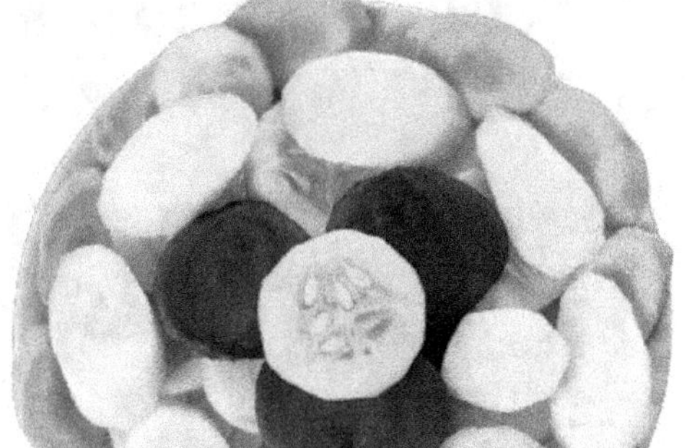

I eat 325 grams of salad of plate-1 just before eating Plate-2.

Plate-1 contains Cucumber, Carrot, Reddish, Beetroot, Cabbage etc. You can take items of salad as per your own choice or seasonal availability.

<h1 style="text-align:center">Plate 2</h1>

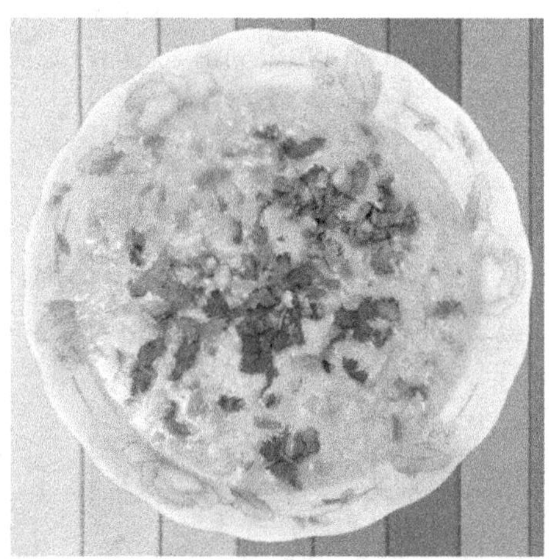

After eating a salad from Plate 1, I eat one bowl of cooked Oats or daliya (Plate 2).

- · **Daliya** is a crushed form of wheat.
- · **Oats** are rich in nutrients and antioxidants. It contains powerful soluble fiber. It helps in managing cholesterol and sugar levels.

18. I Empower First Before Eating or Drinking

As we all know each and everything we eat or drink is basically produced by the Almighty who is the only creator of the universe. Whatever we eat or drink are His creations. So, before consuming them we must remember Him with gratitude and say hearty thanks to Him. I always start eating or drinking with the name of the Almighty. What about you?

Secondly, before eating or drinking, I look at it with respect and repeat in my mind that *each and every particle of the food will remove diseases, weakness, negativity, and abnormality from every cell of my body and it will fill them with perfect health and positive energy.*

While consuming food, I feel that every cell, every tissue, and every organ of my body is being purified and energized by it. I use this powerful technique before drinking or eating anything.

You will be surprised by the results you get in just a few days. It is well known that promises made with faith always work. Just practice this divine technique and get benefits like me. Apart from this, if you continue this, you will also feel connected to the divine power of the universe.

19. Attention!

Learn to drink and eat properly!

Just pay attention to how you eat and drink. Even if you are eating the right food but in the wrong way, it will cause harm rather than benefit. Therefore, there is a need to pay attention to the eating or drinking habits.

Never drink all the water in one go. Drink sip by sip. Similarly, never eat anything in a hurry. Chew each bite thoroughly. If you do not chew your food properly, your intestines will have to do the work of your mouth, which will weaken your digestive power in the future.

Weak digestive power causes many problems like gastric, indigestion, diarrhea, fatigue, stress, weakness, weak immunity, and various serious diseases as well.

While eating, concentrate completely on what you are eating. As far as possible, do not think too much while eating and drinking, and do not remain stressed. Avoid talking while eating. At that time keep your mobile aside also.

> *"Physical fitness is the first requisite of happiness."*
> *– Joseph Pilates*

20. How I Calculate Quantity of Fruits and Salads

Quantity of Fruits = (Your body weight in Kg x 10) grams

= (65 x 10) grams   [Suppose your weight is 65 Kg]

= 650 grams

I eat 650 grams of fruit as my breakfast daily.

Quantity of Salads= (Your body weight Kg x 10) grams

= (65 x 10) grams   [Suppose your weight is 65 Kg]

= 650 grams

Divide this quantity into two parts = 325 gm before lunch (Plate-1) +

325 gm before dinner (Plate-1)

Thus, half of the salads (325 grams) are to be eaten just before lunch and another half (325 grams) is to be eaten just before dinner.

You can calculate the quantity of fruit and salad as per your weight.

I follow the above-mentioned meal plan regularly. However, I cheat once or twice a month. I don't follow any diet plan once or twice a month and eat other foods of my choice that I enjoy.

21. Physical Reforms

What I do

1. I get up 1 hour before the sun rises.
2. After being fresh and performing morning prayer, I do a brisk walk for 30 minutes.
3. Then I exercise for 20 minutes in such a way that I sweat a lot during the exercise.

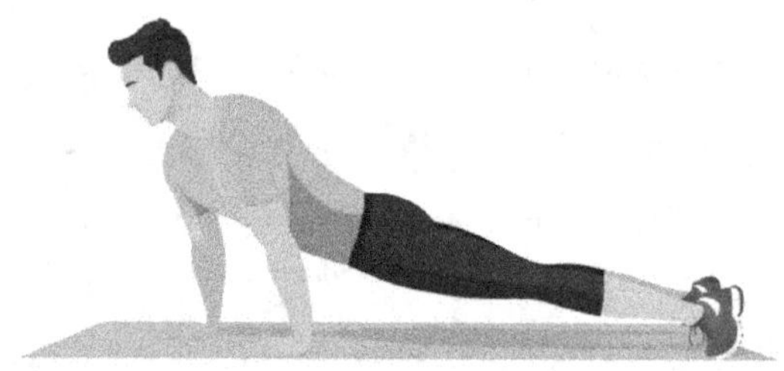

Push-up Exercise

4. I stay barefooted on earth for 10 minutes and do some exercises during this period too.

5. I do breathing exercises (Kapalbhati and Anulom Vilom) for 20 minutes. You can do any breathing exercise of your choice

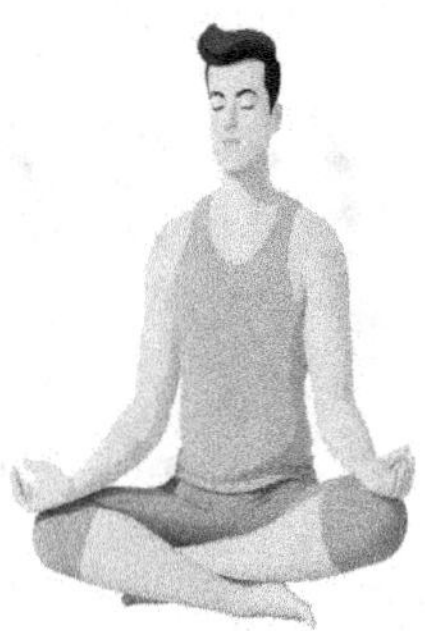

Breathing Exercise and meditation

7. Actually, after exercise and yoga, I do *Shavasana (Corpse Pose)* for 20 minutes with a focus on all major organs of the body one by one. I use an auto-suggestion technique for complete relaxation and self-healing. I do Shavasana along with auto suggestions for healing my body. It gives amazing Results.

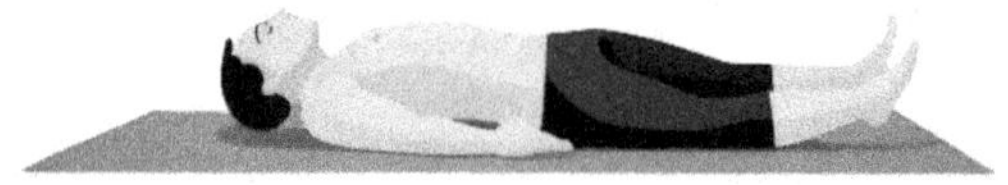

Picture of a Shavasana (Corpse pose)

8. During this process, I give commands to my organs and feel that my organs are getting relaxed, healthy, and full of energy. After some time, I go in half-sleep mode. No matter how much I am tired, I get relaxed soon and feel completely refreshed by doing this Shavasana. This Aasan is amazing and very much beneficial. Its method is explained ahead.

9. I take a bath after relaxation.

> *Optimum nutrition is the medicine of tomorrow."*
> *- Dr. Linus Pauling*

22. Method of Auto Suggestion for Healing and Relaxation

It is well known that our body follows the commands received from the mind. Therefore, I use the below-mentioned method to take benefit of the auto-suggestion technique-

1. Lay down on a flatbed or mat
2. Leave body loose and relaxed
3. Close your eyes and say thanks to the Almighty for your wonderful super body.
4. See with closed eyes and feel that the healing energy of the universe in the form of powerful natural golden rays is showering over your entire body.
5. See that these rays are entering into each and every cell of your body. As a result, diseases, weakness, abnormality, and negativity are being pushed down from cells by these healing rays.
6. These thrown-away diseases are lastly being absorbed by the earth forever.
7. Each and every cell of your body is quickly becoming healthy and full of energy.
8. Now, every cell is happy and enjoying
9. Start seeing body parts with closed eyes from toe to head one by one and say to every part- 'Relax & Energize'
   - Start with Right foot, then left foot, then....
   - Right knee, then left knee
   - Right thigh, then left thigh
   - Private parts one by one
   - Big intestine
   - Small intestine

- · Stomach
- · Liver
- · Pancreas
- · Right kidney, then left kidney, then urinary tract
- · Spine
- · Heart
- · Right lung, then left lung
- · Right hand from fingers to shoulder, then left hand
- · Mouth
- · Right ear, left ear
- · Nose
- · Right eye, left eye
- · Head

During this process when you reach a body part mentioned above and feel that that part is getting relaxed, being healthy, and full of positive energy just keep in mind the below-

i) If you want to *get relaxed* only, say repeatedly to every body part one by one and feel it is "being relaxed....."

ii) *To heal* any organ/part say repeatedly to that body part with

a deep feeling that the organ is - "being healed and energized".

Have a deep and strong feeling that the organ is being healed and energized by the powerful healing rays.

You will learn and understand in the next topic of 'Mental Reform' why and how this Auto Suggestion technique works.

10.   During this process I command organs and feel them becoming relaxed, healthy, and full of energy. After some time, I go into a half-sleep state for a few minutes. No matter how tired I am, by doing this Shavasana my fatigue goes away very quickly and I feel completely refreshed. This asana is very beneficial.

> *"Our bodies are our gardens – our wills are our gardeners."*
>
> *– William Shakespeare*

23. Mental Reforms

This reform is as important as dietary and physical reforms are. The reason behind this is that body and mind are closely connected with each other.

Your body is governed by your mind. That's why the almighty God put the mind at the uppermost part of the body. Whatever you think or you desire, this thought is conveyed to the organ through nerves and the organ follows the desire or the command.

If you want to run, your legs follow this command received from the mind. If you want to clap, your hands follow the command received from the mind. If you want to speak, your mouth follows your commands or thoughts received from the mind.

Thus, you see the body acts as per the thought, the desire, or the command received from the mind. In other words, your body acts as per your thoughts. This is an amazing process and a fact of life as well.

It means, that if your organs receive a command from your mind to be healthy, to be happy, or to be energetic, the same results will be seen in your organs, in your body. Your organs follow the commands in the same way. But to get such results, you will have to send commands with complete faith and focus on that organ.

To master such types of commands and to get the desired results you should have a good understanding of the conscious mind and the subconscious mind.

24. The Conscious Mind and Subconscious Mind

The human mind can be divided into two main components: the Conscious Mind and the Subconscious Mind. These two parts of the mind work together to shape your thoughts, behaviours, and overall well-being.

Conscious Mind: The conscious mind refers to the part of our mental awareness that is currently active and in focus. It is the aspect of our mind that we are consciously aware of at any given moment. This is where we process information, make decisions, and engage in rational thinking. It is associated with our short-term memory and plays a crucial role in our day-to-day activities.

Subconscious Mind: The subconscious mind, on the other hand, is the part of the mind that operates beneath the surface of conscious awareness. It encompasses all the information, memories, and experiences that are not currently in your conscious awareness but can be readily accessed. The subconscious mind is responsible for storing long-term memories, managing automated bodily functions, and influencing our beliefs, habits, and emotions.

In a nutshell, the conscious mind is what you are actively aware of, and it handles logical reasoning and immediate decision-making. In contrast, the subconscious mind operates behind the scenes, storing long-term memories, controlling habits, and influencing emotions and beliefs. Both aspects of the mind work together to shape our thoughts, behaviours, and experiences.

The subconscious mind does not argue. It executes all commands received from the conscious mind. That's why it is said to think positively only.

25. Using the Subconscious Mind for Self-Healing and Well-being

The subconscious mind plays a crucial role in our overall health and energy levels. Here are some ways to harness its power for self-healing and increased vitality:

<u>As you think as you become:</u>

You're what you think. Words that you speak and thoughts that you have in mind, both generate vibrations, a flow of energy in the universe.

You are sending vibrations all the time in the universe because the mind always keeps on thinking. These vibrations spread out in the entire universe in search of the thing of similar energy vibrations and wherever the same is found it is sent towards you. It brings the same vibration that was spread out through your words or thoughts.

Hence, it is truly said that whatever you say or think, the same is brought to you by the universe. So never say or think negatively or badly. Always think and say positive for yourself and for others as well.

As you do see in practical life, people who are always in complaining mode and keep saying negative things, the same they attract. Happiness and prosperity do not come in their life. Negative thoughts attract negative results. Positive thoughts attract positive results. Thus, the choice is yours.

The reason behind it is very clear. It is because Negative thoughts send negative vibrations in the universe and the universe gives the same in return.

On the contrary, if a person always speaks positively and has a passion to achieve his goal, he sends positive vibrations to the universe. The universe searches for the objects/events of the same vibration to give him back.

Thus, whatever thoughts or words you send into the universe the same results are searched for you from the universe.

> *"Happiness is the highest form of health."*
> *– Dalai Lama*

26. How I Manage Diabetes With The Help Of My Subconscious Mind

1. I lay down on a flatbed and I close my eyes.
2. I leave my body loose and relaxed.
3. I take deep breaths and focus on my breathing

   (I see with my closed eyes and feel deeply that...)

4. The healing powers of the universe are showering over my entire body in the form of super-powered cosmic rays.

5. As soon as the healing rays enter into a cell, all diseases, negativity, and abnormality living therein are thrown out and the same are buried down in earth quickly.

6. Each and every cell of my body is being purified and energized.

7. Now, every cell is healthy, happy, and full of life energy

   (I see and feel my digestive parts -intestines, liver, pancreas, etc.)

8. All my digestive internal organs are functioning well and are converting my eaten food into powerful energy.

9. My pancreas is functioning perfectly. It produces insulin as per requirement. Insulin is flowing in the bloodstream and carrying glucose to every cell.
10. In every cell, glucose is converted into energy.
11. Now, every cell possesses enough energy and performs its function perfectly.

12. My every cell is energized, happy, and healthy

13. My every tissue is energized, happy, and healthy

14. My every organ is energized, happy, and healthy

15. My entire body is energized, happy, and healthy

16. A strong positive aura has been created around me

17. My personality has become magnetic, energetic, and universal

18. I am healthy, happy, and prosperous.

19. I sincerely thank the Almighty for all these precious gifts.

If you practice this with full confidence for 20-30 minutes every day, you too will get the desired health like me. Not only your body but also your life will improve dramatically. You can also use this auto-suggestion technique to create abundant wealth. Just practice and get the desired results.

> *"A healthy outside starts from the inside."*
> *– Robert Urich*

27. Spiritual Reform

There is only one God who creates, sustains, and destroys the entire world. He is the master of all of us. He has made man the best creature in the world. Among all living beings, only humans have been given the unique rational power to think and analyze. Love, honesty, purity, and brotherhood are the hallmarks of a human being. These qualities separate humans from animals. Principles of deeds are accepted in all religions. Everyone believes-

1- Good deeds attract good results

2- Bad deeds attract bad results

So, if you are doing evil, be ready to get the same in return. Similarly, if you are practicing good habits, sooner or later, you will certainly get good results.

Acts like lies, deceit, selfishness, theft, dishonesty, hurting others, revenge, hatred, murder, etc. bring humans into the category of animals. Before doing all such bad deeds, a person thinks about them in his mind.

If a person applies all three reforms- Dietary, Physical, and Mental and avoids the Spiritual reform he can hardly be free from diseases, negativity, etc.

Negative thinking releases negative chemicals in the body. Negative chemicals give rise to various diseases in the human body. Every disease of a person's body is the result of his negative thinking.

A person should always be ready for change or improvement. If a person changes his thinking to become natural, i.e. he becomes honest, forgiving to all, and brings love and brotherhood into his life, then his body will once again become healthy and full of energy.

Here are some techniques to practice in daily life to make life peaceful, prosperous, loving, healthy, and energetic-

1. Gratitude- Always say thanks to the Almighty for whatever he has bestowed upon you.
2. Forgive everyone's misdeeds for your peace of mind.
3. Try never to lie. Because one lie forces you to tell many lies.

4. Try to never be dishonest.
5. Every action attracts an equal reaction. So never say bad or do bad.
6. Along with your body, keep your mind pure and holy.
7. Never hate any person. Because everyone gets his own reward for his misdeeds.
8. *Treat others the way you want to be treated.*

All these qualities are divine. If you keep practicing these qualities then your life will become very beautiful, wealthy, and full of happiness.

> *"Physical fitness is the first requisite of happiness."*
> *– Joseph Pilates.*

28. Precious Tips to Make You Healthy & Energetic

1. Eat Homemade foods only; no outside food.
2. Eat only fruits in the morning till noon. Eat salad just before lunch and dinner as per the formula mentioned above.
3. Take a sleep of approximately 7 hours.
4. Do exercise and yoga regularly.
5. Avoid non-veg, dairy products and packaged foods.
6. Do intermittent fasting. Better if you could keep a gap of at least 12 hours between dinner and breakfast.
7. Avoid oily, spicy, and stale foods.
8. Do not talk at the time of eating or drinking. Eat and drink with deep feelings that it will be well digested in your body and will be converted into energy and good health.
9. Use the law of attraction and visualization techniques to make yourself healthier and more energetic.

10. Practice Gratitude. Say thanks to the Almighty for whatever you have

11. Forgive all others to keep your mind peaceful

12. Think only positive; no negative thinking. Be optimistic.

13. Use the technique of auto-suggestion to be healthy- just before sleeping at night and just after you wake in the morning repeat 21 times with deep feeling the same - "I am healthy and energetic"

14. Eat to live, don't live to eat

15. Chilled water decreases the digestive power of the intestines. Hence,

   try not to drink chilled water, even in summer.

16. Learn and Practice the Law of Attraction

17. Must use the superpower of your subconscious mind for health and

   wealth as well.

18. Eat brown rice. Eat bread made of millet in place of wheat.

19. The vibrational frequency of your thoughts spreads out into the universe and searches for things or events of the same frequency for you. Therefore, always think positively for yourself. Think good. Never think negatively. Whatever you think about, you attract to yourself.

If you practice these precious tips in daily life, not only diabetes but other diseases may go away gradually and your body will become healthy, beautiful, and full of energy.

If you can implement four reforms in your life: Dietary, Physical, Mental, and Spiritual; then you will become a real human being full of divine health and happiness with peace of mind.

Dear Reader, one soft reminder again for you- Do not stop your medication to practice the lifestyle explained in this book. Consult your physician first. Do not make a sudden change in eating habits and in living style. You may start the diet plan mentioned above gradually. Observe results. If you get expected results, then go ahead. Go for regular check-ups. Monitor your blood sugar level attentively. If you get sugar level decreases, you may decrease doses of medicines step by step after consultation with your doctor.

Increase your knowledge about natural medicine so that you can make your food your medicine. When you benefit from the natural self-treatment methods described in this book, never forget to share them with others.

<u>Your body is an integrated projection of dietary, physical, mental, and spiritual components. Therefore, all these four input items must be kept in a well-balanced state to get the output of a healthy body.</u>

Always keep in mind the fact mentioned under the title "A Million Dollars Secret" that **metabolic disorders can be corrected by correcting the lifestyle.** This means that diabetes can be reversed through natural therapies, provided this is done under the supervision of a specialist.

May The Almighty bestow His divine blessings on you for a diabetes-free healthy life. I wish you a wonderful happy life. Thank you!

- Shamim Ansari